Nita's Journey Home

P. A. Farrell

Nita's Journey Home

P. A. Farrell

Published by Dr. Patricia A. Farrell, 2026.

NITA'S JOURNEY HOME

First edition. February 7, 2026.

Copyright © 2026 P. A. Farrell.

ISBN: 979-8993739663

Written by P. A. Farrell.

Copyright

The Pocket Companion Series contains:
When Your Mind Won't Stop
After the Loss: Finding Your Way Through Grief
You Are Enough: Rebuilding Your Self-Worth

At the Crossroads: Making Decisions When Nothing Feels Clear

When People Hurt: Navigating Difficult Relationships

When You Feel Stuck: Finding Movement in Hard Times

Books by Patricia A. Farrell, Ph.D.

When You Can't Pour From an Empty Glass: CBT Skills for Exhausted Caregivers

The Little Book on Learning Big Critical Thinking Skills

The Smart Kid's Survival Guide: Making Good Choices in a Confusing World

How to Be Your Own Therapist

It's Not All in Your Head: Anxiety, Depression, Mood Swings and Multiple Sclerosis

Unfiltered: Beneath the noise of our thoughts lies the true narrative of our minds

Unfiltered Again: A behind-the-scenes look at healthcare, medicine and mental health

A Social Security Disability Psychological Claims Handbook: A simple guide to understanding your SSD claim for psychological impairments and unraveling the maze of decision-making

A Social Security Disability Psychological Claims Guidebook for Children's Benefits

The Disability Accessible US Parks in All 50 States: A Comprehensive Guide

Birding in the US NOW!: A birding guide for individuals with disabilities

Chapter 1: The Shaking

The first time it happened, Nita was playing with her doll on the kitchen floor. She was four years old, small for her age, with dark curls that her mother brushed every morning until they shined. The doll had a blue dress that Nita loved to touch, running her tiny fingers over the soft fabric again and again.

Before that day, life was good. It was simple, but it was good. Her father worked at the factory and came home tired but smiling. Her mother kept the house clean and made soup that filled the kitchen with warmth. They lived in three rooms above a butcher shop, and the sounds and smells from the street below were part of Nita's early childhood. Everything seemed fine, just as anyone would hope, but no one suspected that everything would change suddenly.

Nita's world was small but safe. The kitchen where she played. The bedroom she shared with her parents. The front room where her father would sit in his chair after dinner and sometimes let Nita climb onto his lap. She knew the sound of her mother's footsteps, the smell of her father's tobacco, the feeling of being held and loved.

She had a favorite cup, blue with white flowers. Her mother always gave her milk in that cup. And she had a favorite blanket, soft and worn from being carried everywhere. There were routines and rituals that made her feel secure. This was her life, and it was enough.

Then the world went strange. Her arm started to jerk, moving without her wanting it to move. The doll fell from her hand. Nita tried to speak, to call for her mother, but the words wouldn't come. Her whole body began to shake and twist, and she couldn't make it stop. She fell to the floor, her head hitting the worn linoleum.

When Nita woke up, her mother was crying. Her father stood in the doorway, his face white as paper. They spoke in rapid words that Nita didn't understand, their voices sharp with fear. She knew only a little of their language, the old language from the country where they were born. But she knew the fear in their eyes.

"Mother?" she said, reaching up. But her mother pulled back, crossing herself. Making the sign that meant protection. Making the sign that meant danger. Something was terribly wrong and Nita didn't know what it could be.

Her father picked her up gently and carried her to her bed. His hands were shaking. He laid her down and pulled the blanket up to her chin, but he wouldn't look at her face. He kept his eyes on the wall, on the crucifix that hung there, on anything but his little girl.

That night, Nita heard her parents talking in the other room. She couldn't understand most of the words, but she heard one word repeated over and over. A word that made her mother cry harder each time. A word that meant something bad, something wrong. A word that meant Nita was different now.

The shaking came back three days later. This time it happened at dinner. Her fork suddenly fell to the table. The milk spilled across the cloth. Her body jerked and twisted, and she couldn't stop it, couldn't control it. When she woke up this time, she was on the floor and her mouth tasted like blood. She'd bitten her tongue.

Her mother wouldn't touch her. She stood back, her apron clutched in both hands, her lips moving in silent prayer. Her father called for the neighbor woman, Mrs. Farley, who spoke better English. Mrs. Farley came and looked at Nita with sad eyes.

"The child is sick," she told Nita's father in English, so he could understand. "You must take her to the physician."

But Nita's father shook his head. "No physician," he said. "This is not sickness. This is..." He couldn't find the English word. He said something in the old language, something that made Mrs. Farley gasp and step back.

They seemed to be talking about her, but Nita didn't understand. She only knew that something inside her was broken, something she couldn't control. She only knew that her mother wouldn't hold her anymore. Why? What was wrong? She only knew that when she reached for her father's hand, he flinched away.

The shaking came again and again. Sometimes once a day. Sometimes three times. Nita learned to recognize the warning signs. A funny feeling in her stomach. A taste like metal in her mouth. A moment when the world seemed to slow down and get very bright.

But knowing it was coming didn't help. She still couldn't stop it. She still fell. She still woke up confused and sore, with her parents' frightened faces hovering above her.

They stopped letting her play with the other children on the street. They kept her inside, away from windows where neighbors might see. Her mother still fed her and dressed her, but she did it quickly, not looking Nita in the eyes. The brushing of her hair stopped. The bedtime songs stopped. Everything stopped except the fear.

Nita believed what she saw in their eyes. She had made a mistake. That she was bad. That whatever was inside her making her shake and fall was something evil, something that had taken over her body and wouldn't let go.

She was just a little girl who wanted her mother to hold her. Just a little girl who wanted to play with her doll, who didn't understand why her body wouldn't do what she told it to do.

But nobody asked Nita what she wanted. Nobody asked Nita what she felt. Nobody explained anything to her in words she could understand. They just watched her with fearful eyes and whispered words she couldn't quite hear.

And the shaking kept coming, again and again, until it became the only thing Nita knew about herself. She was the girl who shook. She was the girl who fell. She was the girl who made her parents afraid.

Chapter 2: The Visitors

The visitors started coming on a Tuesday evening. Nita was in her room, sitting on her bed with her doll, when she heard the knock at the door. Heavy footsteps in the hallway. Voices speaking the old language, low and serious.

Her father came to get her. His face was set in hard lines, like he'd made a decision he didn't want to make. "Come, Nita," he said. Not in English this time. He spoke to her in the old language now, as if the English had been a luxury they could no longer afford.

In the kitchen, three people waited. An old man with a long gray beard, wearing black clothes and carrying a bag. A woman with a scarf tied tight around her head, her lips moving in silent prayer. And another man, younger, holding a book bound in cracked leather.

They looked at Nita with eyes that weren't afraid, exactly, but wary. Like she was a dog that might bite. The old man with the beard stepped forward and said something to her father. Her father nodded and stepped back, leaving Nita alone in the center of the room.

The old man opened his bag and took out a bottle of water. He sprinkled it on Nita's head, speaking words in a language even older than the one her parents spoke. The water was cold. It ran down her forehead and dripped onto her dress. Nita shivered.

The younger man opened his book and began to read. His voice rose and fell in a rhythm that would have been soothing if it weren't for the fear in the room. The woman with the scarf joined in, her voice high and thin. Nita's mother stood in the corner, weeping quietly.

They prayed over Nita for hours. The old man touched her forehead, her hands, her feet. He spoke words that were supposed to make the evil go away. Words that were supposed to fix whatever was broken inside her. But Nita felt the same. Nothing changed except that she got tired and her legs hurt from standing still for so long.

When the visitors finally left, her father gave them money. Nita saw him counting out the bills with shaking hands. Money they didn't have. Money that should have bought food or paid the rent. But he gave it to them anyway, because they had promised to help his daughter.

The next day, the shaking came anyway. Nita was eating breakfast when the familiar feeling started in her stomach. The metal taste. The brightness. She tried to say something, to warn them, but it was too late. Her body jerked and twisted. The bowl of oatmeal crashed to the floor. She fell after it.

When she woke up, her mother was crying again. Not the quiet tears from before, but deep, wrenching sobs that shook her whole body. The visitors hadn't worked. The prayers hadn't worked. Nita was still broken.

More visitors came. Different ones this time. A woman who burned herbs that made the whole house smell like smoke. A man who tied a red string around Nita's wrist and told her never to take it off. Another old man who made her drink bitter tea that made her stomach hurt.

Each visitor brought their own methods, their own rituals, their own promises. Some were gentle, speaking softly as they anointed Nita with oils that smelled like strange flowers. Others were fierce, shouting in languages Nita didn't understand, making dramatic gestures meant to drive out whatever darkness they believed possessed her.

One woman insisted Nita sleep with a small cloth bag under her pillow, filled with herbs and stones and a piece of paper with words written in an alphabet Nita had never seen. Nita obeyed, though the bag was lumpy and uncomfortable. She would have done anything if it meant the shaking would stop, if it meant her mother would hold her again.

Another visitor, a thin man with darting eyes, said that Nita needed to be cleansed by ice. He filled the bathtub with water so cold it made Nita gasp, made her chest feel tight. He held her in that freezing water while he chanted, and Nita cried from the cold and the fear and the confusion of not understanding why this was happening to her.

Her mother stood in the doorway during these sessions, her face pale, her hands clutching her apron. She never stopped the visitors. Never said this was too much, that Nita was just a little girl who needed comfort, not ceremonies. She'd given up her maternal protectiveness to fear and superstition, and Nita felt that abandonment more keenly than any physical discomfort the visitors inflicted.

Each time, her father paid money. Each time, they promised it would work. Each time, the shaking came back anyway.

Nita started to feel like she wasn't a person anymore. She was a problem to be solved. A thing to be fixed. People touched her and prayed over her and gave her things to drink, but nobody talked to her. Nobody asked her if she was scared. Nobody told her it would be okay.

The worst was the night they brought in the group. Seven people, all dressed in black, all carrying candles. They made Nita lie on the floor in the middle of a circle. They stood around her, chanting and swaying. The candlelight made strange shadows on the walls. Nita closed her eyes tight, wishing she could disappear.

They said she had something inside her. Something bad. Something that needed to be forced out. They shouted at it, commanded it to leave. Their voices got louder and louder until Nita wanted to cover her ears. But she'd been told to lie still, to not move, so she did.

When it was over, they told her father that the thing inside her was very strong. It would take more sessions. More prayers. More money. Her father, exhausted and desperate, agreed to everything.

But Nita knew the truth, even at four years old. There was nothing inside her. There was just her body, doing something she couldn't control. There was just her, scared and confused, wanting someone to make it stop.

The visitors came and went for weeks. Months. Each one with their own rituals, their own promises, their own prices. And through it all, Nita just wanted to be held. She wanted her mother to brush her hair again. She wanted her father to smile at her the way he used to.

But those days were gone. Now there were only the visitors, the prayers, the fear, and the shaking that never stopped, no matter how many people tried to drive it away.

Chapter 3: The Physician

Dr. Farley was old, with hands that shook almost as much as Nita's body did during her spells. He'd been practicing medicine in their town for forty years, mostly seeing people for colds and broken bones and babies being born. He wasn't the kind of physician who dealt with problems like Nita's.

But he was Mrs. Farley's husband, and she'd finally convinced Nita's father to bring the child in. "Just let him look," she'd said. "What harm can it do? You've tried everything else."

One morning, after another night of visitors and prayers that hadn't worked, Nita's father wrapped her in a blanket and carried her to Dr. Farley's office. It was above the drugstore on Division Street, reached by a narrow stairway that smelled of tobacco.

The office was small and cluttered. Books were piled on every surface. The examination table was covered with cracked leather that was cold against Nita's legs when her father set her down. There was a chart on the wall showing the inside of a person's body, all the organs and bones labeled in tiny letters.

The physician looked at Nita for a long time. Not with fear like her parents. Not with the determined certainty of the visitors who'd tried to fix her. Just... looking. Studying. His watery blue eyes moved from her face to her hands to her feet and back again.

"Tell me what happens," he said to Nita's father in English, speaking slowly so he would understand. "Tell me exactly what you see."

Her father struggled with the words. His English was poor, made worse by his exhaustion and fear. But Dr. Farley was patient. He asked questions. He listened. He wrote notes in a leather notebook with cramped, careful handwriting.

Then the physician did something none of the visitors had done. He talked to Nita. Not at her, not around her, but to her. He knelt down so his face was level with hers.

"Does it hurt?" he asked gently.

Nita didn't know how to answer. Sometimes it hurt, the falling and the hitting. Sometimes it didn't. Sometimes she just felt tired and confused when it was over. She shrugged, a small movement that made her father shift nervously behind her.

"Do you feel it coming?" Dr. Farley asked. "Before it happens, do you feel something different?"

This question Nita could answer. She nodded. The metal taste. The funny feeling. The brightness. Yes, she felt it coming. Not that it helped. She still couldn't stop it.

Dr. Farley examined her. He looked in her eyes with a small light. He listened to her heart. He tapped her knees with a little rubber hammer and watched her leg kick out. He was gentle, but Nita was still scared. She'd had enough of people touching her, doing things to her, trying to fix her.

When he was done, Dr. Farley stood up slowly, his knees creaking. He went to his desk and sat down heavily. For a long time, he just looked at his notes. Nita's father waited, standing by the door, his cap clutched in both hands.

"This is not possession," Dr. Farley finally said. "This is not evil spirits or demons. This is illness. Sickness of the mind, perhaps. Or something wrong in the brain that makes her body do these things."

Nita's father didn't understand all the words, but he understood enough. He shook his head violently. "No," he said.

"Not sick. Not crazy. She is..." He couldn't find the English words for what he wanted to say.

Dr. Farley sighed. He was too old and too tired to argue with superstition. He'd seen it before, this refusal to accept that sometimes the body just breaks in ways we don't understand. He'd seen families pour their money into prayers and rituals rather than face the harder truth.

Some families were so desperate that they took their child to shrines abroad in Asia, Africa, and Egypt. Each time they hoped they would find a cure for what was affecting their child but there was no cure anywhere. One family even sought out a magical witch doctor they had heard about and scoured the countryside until they found him. He made a concoction and gave it to their child, who immediately became sick to their stomach and developed a high fever, but nothing changed.

Still, they searched in hopes that there would be someone who could cure their child. They asked everyone they knew and sent letters to important religious figures asking for prayers or amulets. For all their efforts, they found nothing. Bags of trinkets, amulets, and secret messages that were to be whispered under the moon at night were left with them. They tried everything to no avail.

In the small town where Nita lived, the doctor made a life-changing determination. "She needs to go to the hospital," he said. "The state hospital. They have physicians there who understand these things. They can help her." There was no other hope for the couple and their daughter needed to go where Dr. Farley indicated.

The state hospital. Everyone in town knew what that meant. It was the place for people whose minds had broken. The place for the violent, the dangerous, the unsalvageable. It was fifty miles away, a sprawling campus of solid stone, walled buildings surrounded by high barbed wire fences. People went there and sometimes they never came back.

Nita's father went pale. "No," he said again. "Please, no."

But Dr. Farley was already writing on an official form. "I must report this," he said, not unkindly. "It's the law. A child with this condition... she needs proper care. Care you cannot give her at home."

He handed the form to Nita's father. "Take this to the courthouse," he said. "They will make the arrangements."

Nita didn't understand what was happening. She only knew that her father's face had gone from fearful to something else. Something worse. A kind of defeated sadness that made his shoulders slump and his hands shake as he took the paper.

They walked home in silence. Nita's father carried her, but differently than before. As if she were already gone. As if she were already someone else's problem, someone else's responsibility.

That night, Nita heard her parents crying together in the living room. She'd heard her mother cry many times. But her father's tears were new, harsh sounds that seemed torn from somewhere deep inside him. Sounds of a man who had tried everything and failed.

Over the next three weeks, Nita watched her parents prepare for her departure in small, heartbreaking ways. Her mother washed and mended Nita's clothes with extra care, her hands shaking as she sewed. Her father built a small wooden box to hold Nita's few belongings, working late into the night in the small space by the window, the sound of his hammer echoing through the rooms.

They didn't talk about where Nita was going. They couldn't seem to say the words out loud. But Nita knew something terrible was coming. She could feel it in the way they looked at her now—with a kind of desperate sadness, trying to memorize her face, as if she were already gone.

The night before the car came, her mother held Nita for the first time in months. Really held her, not just touching her out of necessity. She rocked Nita in her arms and sang an old song from the country where she'd been born. Nita didn't understand all the words, but she understood the grief in them. The song was about children who went away and never came home.

Her father stood in the doorway, watching. His face was wet with tears he didn't bother to wipe away. Nita had never seen her father cry before. It scared her more than the seizures ever had.

The car came and took Nita away.

Chapter 4: The Hospital

The state hospital looked like a small town. Gray field stone buildings spread across acres of lawn, connected by concrete paths. Trees lined the roads. There was even a church with a white steeple. From a distance, it might have looked peaceful. Beautiful, even.

Up close, you noticed other things. The heavy screens and bars on the windows. The high fence around the property. The way some of the windows on the upper floors were painted over so you couldn't see in or out. The men in white coats who walked the paths, watching.

Nita arrived in a black car with a woman from the county who smiled too much and spoke in a voice that was too bright. Her father hadn't come. Her mother hadn't come. They'd said goodbye at home, awkward and brief, her mother crossing herself one more time, her father turning away so Nita wouldn't see his face.

The woman from the county took Nita to Building C, Ward 2. The children's ward. Inside, it smelled like disinfectant and something else, something Nita couldn't name. Fear, maybe. Or sadness so old it had seeped into the walls.

A nurse met them at the desk. She was young, with red hair pulled back from her face. She looked at Nita with tired eyes and took a clipboard from the county woman.

"Another one," the nurse said, signing the papers. Not cruel, just matter-of-fact. Children came here all the time. Children whose families couldn't or wouldn't keep them. Children whose minds or bodies didn't work the way they should.

The county woman left quickly, her heels clicking on the green linoleum. Nita wanted to run after her, back to the car, back home. But the nurse's hand was firm on her shoulder.

"Come on, then," the nurse said. "Let's get you settled."

The ward was a long room with beds lined up on both sides. Twenty beds, maybe more. Some were empty. Some had children in them, lying still or rocking back and forth or making sounds that weren't quite words. The windows were high up on the walls, letting in light but not much else.

The nurse took Nita to a bed near the middle. The metal frame was painted white, but the paint was chipping. The mattress was thin and covered with a gray blanket. There was a small metal locker beside it with a dent in the side.

"This is yours," the nurse said. "You'll sleep here. You'll keep your things in the locker. Breakfast is at seven, lunch at noon, dinner at five. If you follow the rules, you won't have any problems." Nita wondered what rules the nurse meant. There hadn't been rules like this at home. Now she was expected to follow rules.

Nita didn't know what the rules were. She stood by the bed, small and frightened, clutching the paper bag that held her one dress, her nightgown, and her doll.

The nurse looked at her for a moment, and something in her face softened. "You'll be all right," she said, but she didn't sound convinced. Then she was gone, her shoes squeaking on the floor, off to deal with the next child, the next problem, the endless stream of broken lives that came through these doors.

Nita sat on the edge of her bed. She didn't know what else to do. Around her, the other children paid her no attention. A girl in the next bed was singing to herself, the same note over and over. A boy across the room was hitting his head against the wall with a steady rhythm. No one stopped him.

That first night, Nita cried. But quietly, into her thin pillow, so the nurses wouldn't hear. She didn't know if crying was against the rules. She didn't want to find out. And there were other sounds, too, that she couldn't make out, but she figured it might be someone who had broken the rules.

The days began to blur together. Wake up when the bell rang. Stand by your bed for inspection. Line up to eat breakfast in the cafeteria. Sit in the dayroom. Eat lunch. Sit some more. Eat dinner. Go to bed. Every day the same. There was never any time or any indication that play was a part of her routine. Even going outside was carefully controlled when suggested. At home, Nita's mother used to take her for walks on sunny days, but here, even if the sun was shining bright, they were kept indoors.

A physician saw Nita once, maybe twice in those first weeks. He had a clipboard and asked questions she didn't understand. He made notes. He prescribed medicine that came in little paper cups, pills that made her feel fuzzy and distant from herself.

The shaking still came. When it did, the nurses would come and hold her down until it stopped. Sometimes they put her in a different room, a small room with padding on the walls. They called it the quiet room. There was nothing quiet about it. Nita could hear other children screaming from similar rooms down the hall. No one paid attention and no one ever came when someone screamed. Screaming seemed to be a part of the environment. Once she did see a child taken out in a strange-looking jacket that had buckles in the back. The child was trying to bite someone and they were holding him down, at least four of them. She never saw that child again.

Weeks turned into months. Months turned into years. Nita waited for her mother and father to come get her. She waited by the window during visiting hours, watching the parking lot. But no one came. Not that week. Not that month. Not ever. No letters, no cards, no communication whatsoever from anyone in her family, her neighbors, or her school.

She learned that this was her home now. This bed. This ward. These walls. The other children didn't leave either, except when they got too old and were moved to the adult buildings or to another hospital in some other part of the state. The hospital was a world unto itself, and Nita was now a part of it.

She learned to be a patient. To line up when told. To take her medicine without complaint. To keep her head down and not cause trouble. To accept that this was all there was, all there would ever be.

She was four years old when she arrived. By the time she was five, she could barely remember her parents' faces. By the time she was six, home was just a dream she'd had once, growing fainter with each passing day.

But some memories persisted, fragments that would surface at unexpected moments. The smell of her mother's cooking. The sound of her father's laugh. The feeling of being held. These memories were painful because they reminded Nita of what she'd lost. Eventually, she learned to push them away, to not think about the before times. It hurt too much.

The hospital had its own cruel kindnesses. A nurse who would sometimes sneak an extra cookie at snack time. An orderly who knew magic tricks and would perform them for the children when he had a spare moment. A janitor who would hum songs while he mopped, cheerful tunes that briefly lifted the oppressive atmosphere of the ward.

But these moments of light only made the darkness more apparent. For every kind nurse, there were two who were burned out, exhausted, going through the motions with no energy left for compassion. For every magic trick, there were hours of sitting on hard benches in the day room with nothing to do, nowhere to go, no one who cared.

Nita learned the unspoken rules quickly. Don't ask for things. Don't complain. Don't cry where anyone can see you. Don't form attachments. Don't hope. Hope was dangerous in a place like this. Hope could break you more thoroughly than resignation ever would.

The seasons changed outside the high windows, but inside the ward, every day felt the same. Summer, winter, spring, and fall only brought small changes in temperature. The real way to tell time was by who arrived and who left. New children came in, scared and confused. Older children moved to adult wards or sometimes died. People came and went all the time, reminding everyone that this was a place where people were kept, not where they truly lived.

Chapter 5: The Years

Time in the hospital didn't move the same way it did outside. There were no seasons, really. The same 25-watt incandescent bulbs burned overhead, whether it was summer or winter. The same walls surrounded Nita whether she was ten or twenty or forty.

As she grew, her body changed. She got taller, then stopped growing. She became a teenager, though no one celebrated her birthdays. She became an adult, at least in years. But her mind stayed young, trapped in the child she'd been when she arrived.

How could she grow up? Everything was decided for her. When to wake. When to eat. What to wear. Where to go. The nurses told her what to do, and Nita did it. That was all she knew. That was all she'd ever been allowed to know.

She was moved from the children's ward to the women's ward when she turned eighteen. Different building, different bed, but the same routine. The same emptiness. The same absence of choice.

The worst part was the pain in her feet. It started when she was in her thirties and got worse every year. A deep, burning ache that made walking hard. The nurses said it was arthritis, gave her pills that didn't help much. And someone even suggested that the man who came occasionally with a huge box full of special shoes might have ones to fit her. They called them orthopedic shoes and the hospital would grudgingly pay for them if the pain were unbearable.

But Nita's mind, still like a child's, couldn't understand arthritis. She just knew her feet hurt, burned, throbbed, and felt

21

wrong. She began to imagine her feet were talking to her, telling her things and complaining about walking on the hard floors all day.

When she mentioned this to a nurse, trying to explain the pain in the only way that made sense to her, the nurse wrote it down in her chart. Auditory hallucinations, the chart said. Hearing voices. The physician increased her medication.

The pills made her foggy. Made it hard to think. But the pain in her feet didn't go away, and neither did the feeling that they were trying to tell her something. So Nita learned not to mention it anymore. She learned to keep quiet about a lot of things.

The seizures, the shaking that had brought her here in the first place, came less often as she got older. Sometimes months would pass without one. But the hospital didn't let her go. She'd been diagnosed with mental illness. She'd been committed. This was her life now, for better or worse.

Years passed. Decades. The nurses who'd been young when Nita arrived grew old and retired. New nurses came, just as tired, just as overwhelmed. Nita became one of the fixtures of the ward, someone who'd been there so long that nobody questioned it anymore.

She never received a letter. Never got a phone call. Never had a visitor. Not once in all those years. If her parents had lived or died, if she had siblings who wondered about her, if anyone in the world outside these walls remembered she existed, she didn't know. No one told her. No one thought to ask if she wanted to know.

Sometimes, late at night, lying in her narrow bed, Nita would try to remember her mother's face. The way she used to brush Nita's hair before everything went wrong. The songs she used to sing. But the memories were faded now, worn thin like an old photograph left too long in the sun.

She had a friend for a while, another patient named Marie who'd been in a car accident that had damaged her brain. Marie was kind. She and Nita would sit together in the day room, not talking much, just being together. It was nice to have someone.

But then Marie died one winter, pneumonia taking her in just three days. They came and took her bed away. Put another patient in it within a week. And Nita learned another lesson about life in the hospital: don't get too attached. Everyone leaves eventually, one way or another.

The television in the dayroom showed her that the world was changing. Color TV replaced black and white. Hemlines went up and down. Presidents changed. Wars were fought and ended. The moon landing. Computers. Cell phones. The world moved forward, but inside the hospital, time stood still.

Nita learned the rhythms of institutional life. She knew which nurses were kind and which were harsh. She knew which patients to avoid and which meals were the least awful. She knew how to make herself small and quiet so she wouldn't be noticed, wouldn't be trouble.

She learned that crying didn't help. That asking questions made the nurses impatient. That the world was divided into people who gave orders and people who followed them, and she would always, always be in the second category.

Her hair went gray. Her face developed lines. Her hands grew gnarled with arthritis. She was an old woman now, though her mind was still that of a confused little girl trying to understand why her parents had sent her away.

Sixty-five years passed. Sixty-five years of the same walls, the same routine, the same emptiness. Sixty-five years of waiting for someone to come get her, to take her home, to tell her it had all been a mistake.

But nobody came. And slowly, painfully, Nita stopped waiting.

There were small moments of kindness over the years. A nurse named Rita who would sometimes brush Nita's hair gently, the way her mother used to. An orderly named James who always made sure Nita got the better of the dinner choices when he could. These tiny gestures of humanity in an otherwise dehumanizing place meant everything.

But they never lasted. Rita retired. James got transferred to another building. The kind people came and went, replaced by new staff who saw Nita as just another patient in a never-ending stream of them. Each time someone kind left, it was like losing a small piece of home all over again.

The holidays were the hardest. Christmas especially. The hospital would put up decorations—a plastic tree in the dayroom, paper snowflakes taped to the windows. Other patients would get visits from family, cards in the mail, packages wrapped in bright paper. Nita would watch from her corner, hands folded in her lap, trying not to want what she could never have.

Christmas gifts came from a traveling salesman's trunk and included sweaters, slippers, and pajamas. No one could choose the color or what they received. The nurse picked out everything and handed it out after a volunteer wrapped each gift in a single piece of paper.

The sweaters and pajamas were thin, and the slippers barely covered your feet. Anyone with larger or wider feet still had to squeeze into whatever was given. If they refused, they were seen as a problem and could be sent to the quiet room.

No one wanted to go to the quiet room because it meant being completely alone, with no one checking on you. There was a bucket in the corner for your use, but no way to wash your hands, and only a thin mat on the floor to lie on. There was no blanket, no chair, nothing else. Meals were almost forgotten, and patients in quiet rooms sometimes begged for food. Nita saw one woman beg at the small window in the door for coffee or bread, but everyone ignored her. It was as if she didn't exist.

Sometimes people in the quiet room died suddenly, and then the room would be opened. Nita once saw a woman's legs sticking out from the quiet room before staff came with a gurney to take her away. They didn't hurry, and the woman lay there for hours because they couldn't find a gurney on the unit. That wasn't unusual since when one of the patients had an infection that needed to be washed frequently, the nurse had to use a vegetable tray from the refrigerator because they had no basins on the unit. She also found out that the oxygen unit was empty when they tried to use it to revive a patient who had just swallowed batteries. As his face turned purple, the nurse screamed for help and someone had to run to another unit to bring back an oxygen mask. Supplies were always deficient.

One year, when Nita was in her forties, a volunteer group came to sing carols. They stood in the hallway, their voices bright and cheerful, singing about home and family and love. Nita had to excuse herself, shuffle back to her bed, and press her face into the pillow to muffle the sobs that came from somewhere deep inside. Yes, Nita still knew how to cry but she tried to suppress it whenever it rose up.

A nurse found her there an hour later, still crying. The nurse—one of the new ones who didn't know Nita well—made a note in the chart. Depression, it said. Adjusted medication. But it wasn't depression that made Nita cry. It was grief. Grief for the life she'd never had. Grief for the seventy Christmases she'd spent alone.

Chapter 6: The Workshop

The workshop was in the basement of Building D. It smelled like glue and cardboard and the sweat of people working in a room with no windows. This was where some of the higher-functioning patients went during the day to do piecework for local businesses. The hospital had contracts with these companies that paid pennies for units made by patients sitting at long tables and assembling small items all day long.

Nita had been coming here for twenty years. Five days a week, nine to three, with a break for lunch. The work was simple: pushing small rectangular sponges into cardboard backing cards. The cards would be sold around the country in small and large stores. People would use them to clean their kitchen counters, never knowing they'd been assembled by patients in a state hospital.

The supervisor, Mr. Bowers, was a small man with glasses that were always sliding down his nose. He wasn't cruel, but he wasn't particularly kind either. He was just a man doing a job, managing a workforce of people who'd been forgotten by the world outside.

Nita was good at the work. Her hands might be gnarled with arthritis, but they were steady. She could push sponges into cards faster than almost anyone else in the workshop. She took pride in this, in being useful, in doing something well.

At the end of each week, Mr. Bowers would give them their pay. It wasn't much. The contract the hospital had with the business paid by the piece, and after the hospital took its cut for room and board, which they weren't allowed to do by law but did anyway, what was left was pitiful. Nita made about forty dollars a month. Forty dollars for six hours a day, five days a week.

But it was hers. Her money. The only thing in the world that belonged to her. She kept it in an envelope in her locker, counted it sometimes just to feel like she had something, even though counting was difficult because she had very little schooling in the hospital. School in the hospital, in fact, was little more than coloring for hours.

The other workers in the shop were a mixed group. There was Harold, who'd been a lawyer before his breakdown. He never spoke about what had happened, just sat at his table pushing sponges with the same precise care he'd probably once used to draft legal documents.

There was Betty, who laughed at things no one else found funny and sometimes forgot to push the sponges, just stacked them in neat piles until Mr. Bowers noticed and redirected her. No one blamed her because she had great difficulty breathing because of the medication that had caused permanent damaging changes in her body's breathing apparatus, her diaphragm. Just trying to breathe was an effort for Betty. Along with the breathing difficulty, came the fact that she couldn't stop her mouth from moving in peculiar ways as well.

Then there was Tom, who'd been in the hospital since he was a teenager and was now in his fifties. He had a system for everything, counted each sponge before he used it, arranged his cards in perfect rows. If anything disrupted his system, he would shut down completely, rocking in his chair until Mr. Bowers helped him start over. No one paid any attention to him as he went through his motions or had one of his meltdowns.

Nita didn't talk much to the others. She'd learned that conversations could be dangerous. Say the wrong thing and it might end up in your chart. Show too much emotion and they might adjust your medication. Better to keep your head down and just work.

But there was a rhythm to the work that Nita found soothing. Pick up a card. Push. Press sponge. Set aside. Repeat. Repeat. Repeat. Her hands knew what to do without her having to think about it. Her mind could wander, but it had little to wander to because she had little interaction with any environment outside the hospital. There were never any trips that she was taken on to go to the local mall or a shopping center or even a supermarket.

Sometimes she imagined that someone would buy one of her sponges. Maybe a woman with a family, with a kitchen that smelled like cooking instead of disinfectant. Maybe that woman would use the sponge Nita had made and never know that someone who'd been locked away from the world for sixty-five years had touched it, had put it together with care.

It was a strange connection to the outside world—weak and one-sided, but still something. These thoughts didn't come often as she sat each day, mindlessly assembling sponges and cards. Sometimes, when someone had a meltdown and work stopped because of a fight, it was almost a relief. Of course, fights meant someone would end up in the quiet room.

Mr. Bowers appreciated Nita's reliability. She was never late. Never caused problems. Never had outbursts or refused to work. Whenever she was sick, she wanted to go to work and fought to go to work and never wanted to stay in her bed to get better.

In his quarterly reports to the hospital administration, he always marked her as an exemplary worker.

But it didn't matter. Those reports just went into a file. Nobody read them or cared that Nita was reliable or took pride in her work. She was just another patient, another number, someone the state paid for and the administration benefited from. The administrators had special apartments on the top floor, furnished with antiques collected by the hospital over the years. They even had their own cook, and their meals never came from the big vats in the hospital kitchen.

But Nita didn't know that. She thought that if she just worked hard enough, was good enough, quiet enough, maybe something would change. Maybe someone would notice. Maybe someone would say she'd done well, that she could go home now. *Home* was a word that was almost a strange language to her now.

She'd been thinking that for sixty-five years. The hope never quite died, even when all evidence suggested it should.

The workshop was her world now. Nine to three, five days a week. Sponges and cardboard. The squeak of Mr. Bowers's shoes on the tile floor. The smell of industrial adhesives. The quiet satisfaction of a job done well.

Sometimes Nita would calculate in her head how many sponges she'd carded. Thousands, certainly. Tens of thousands, probably. If you lined them all up, would they stretch across the whole hospital grounds? Would they reach the fence? Would they reach beyond the fence to the town, to the world outside that Nita had stopped believing she'd ever see again?

The work gave her something the hospital rarely provided: a sense of purpose. In the ward, she was just taking up space, consuming resources, existing. But in the workshop, she was producing something. Creating something. It didn't matter that it was just sponges on cards. It mattered that her hands made them, that her effort had a tangible result.

Sometimes Mr. Bowers would comment on her work. "Good job, Nita," he'd say, examining a stack of her finished cards. "Very neat. Very consistent." These small words of praise were precious to her. She'd replay them in her mind later, in the long empty hours of the evening, holding onto them like treasures.

She fantasized sometimes about meeting someone who'd bought one of her sponges. She'd imagine walking up to them and in this fantasy, she was somehow free, somehow out in the world and saying, "I made that." She imagined them being impressed, grateful. She imagined mattering to someone, anyone, even in this small way.

But it was just a fantasy. Nita knew she would never meet those people. She would never leave this place. The sponges would go out into the world, into kitchens, and bathrooms and lives she could only imagine, and she would stay here, pushing sponges into cards, day after day after day, until she was too old or too sick to work anymore.

It wasn't much of a life. But it was the only one Nita had ever known.

Chapter 7: The Quiet Room

The quiet room was not quiet at all. That was the first thing anyone learned. It was a small room with walls covered in material softer than the concrete behind it, but now gray with age and stained in ways you didn't want to think about. The door was heavy and had a small window with wire mesh.

When they put you in the quiet room, you could hear everything. The screams from other rooms. The footsteps of nurses in the hallway. The clanging of food carts. The sound of your own breathing, loud in your ears. But you couldn't make noise yourself. That was the point. The quiet room was for patients who needed to calm down, who needed to be removed from the general population.

Nita knew the quiet room well—too well. She had been there more times than she could count. Sometimes it was for good reasons, like when she had seizures and needed a safe place to recover. But often, it was for reasons that seemed small and unimportant.

Like the time with the spoon.

It was lunchtime in the cafeteria. Nita had been served her meal—some kind of gray meat, watery vegetables, and a roll that was hard as a rock. She was hungry. She'd been looking forward to lunch all morning, thinking about it while she carded sponges in the workshop.

She was halfway through eating when an orderly came by, the new guy with the crew cut and the too-tight uniform. He was checking trays, making sure no one was hoarding food. Hoarding things like bread or fruit juice meant somebody was going to try to make alcohol on the unit. When he got to Nita's table, he decided she'd had enough.

"Give me the tray," he said.

Nita looked down at her food. She wasn't done. She was still hungry. Her feet hurt from standing all morning, and she needed to eat. She shook her head.

"I said give me the tray." His voice was harder now. He wasn't asking anymore.

Something in Nita snapped. Maybe it was hunger. Maybe it was the pain in her feet. Maybe it was sixty-five years of having everything taken from her, never being allowed to say no, and never having any control over her life. Nita threw the spoon at him; it wasn't a hard throw. The spoon bounced off his chest and clattered to the floor. It didn't hurt him. Didn't even leave a mark. But that didn't matter.

Two more orderlies appeared from nowhere. They grabbed Nita's arms, hauled her out of her seat. She didn't resist. She knew better than to resist. One of the patients had gotten her arm broken that way. But her tray fell to the floor anyway, her lunch spilling across the tile floor.

They took her to the quiet room. Locked the door behind her. Left her there for the rest of the day and into the evening. No dinner. No bathroom breaks. Just Nita and the walls and the sounds of the hospital filtering through the door.

By the time they let her out, she was dizzy with hunger and humiliation. The head nurse, Mrs. Sauers, was waiting for her.

"That kind of behavior is unacceptable," Mrs. Sauers said. "You're lucky we don't report this to the physician. He could increase your medication. Or give you an injection. Is that what you want?"

Nita shook her head. That wasn't what she wanted. She just wanted to finish her lunch. She wanted the pain to stop. More than anything, she wanted to be treated like a person, not just a problem to be managed.

But she couldn't say any of that. So she just kept her head down and mumbled an apology.

After that, whenever anything went wrong on the ward, they looked at Nita first. A patient got agitated? Must have been something Nita did. Someone's belongings went missing? Check Nita's locker. An argument broke out in the dayroom? Put Nita in the quiet room until things settled down.

It didn't matter that Nita was usually innocent. It didn't matter that she kept to herself, tried to stay out of trouble. She'd thrown that spoon. She'd shown that she could be difficult. And in a place like this, where control was everything, difficulty was the worst sin you could commit.

The quiet room became as familiar as her own bed. The patterns in the wall. The scratch marks on the door where someone had tried to claw their way out. The way the light fixture hummed, a sound that got inside your head and wouldn't leave.

Nita learned to endure it. What choice did she have? She learned to sit very still, to breathe slowly, to wait until they decided she'd been punished enough. She learned that fighting back only made things worse. She learned that in here, justice didn't exist. Only power.

The quiet room taught her other lessons too. It taught her that her feelings didn't matter. That her hunger, her pain, her fear, her need for fairness—none of it counted for anything. It taught her that she was less than human in the eyes of the institution. A problem to be managed, not a person to be respected.

Sometimes, in those long hours alone, Nita would talk to herself. Quiet conversations that no one else could hear. She'd tell herself stories about a different life, a different Nita who lived in a house with people who loved her. She'd imagine that other Nita eating meals at a table, sleeping in a soft bed, making choices about her own life.

These fantasies kept her sane in the quiet room. They reminded her that somewhere inside, despite everything, she was still a person with desires and dreams. Even if those dreams would never come true, even if that other life was impossible, holding onto them kept some small part of her alive.

The staff never understood this. To them, Nita was a management problem. A patient who occasionally needed to be isolated for the good of the ward. They didn't see the human cost of the quiet room. Didn't see how it eroded dignity, crushed spirit, reinforced the message that Nita was worthless.

Or maybe they did see it and just didn't care. Maybe after years of working in a place like this, you had to stop caring. Once they began getting that $1.25 lunch for employees, it was all over. They had to stop seeing the patients as fully human. Otherwise, how could you lock them in rooms? How could you take away their food? How could you punish them for the smallest infractions while calling it treatment?

And she had none.

Chapter 8: The Evaluation

The people from the outside agency came on a Tuesday morning in early spring. Nita was seventy-four years old, though she couldn't have told you that if you'd asked. Time had lost meaning long ago.

There were three of them: a young woman with a clipboard and caring eyes, a man with gray hair who looked tired, and another woman who was older and walked with a cane. They set up in the conference room, the one that was usually locked, and started calling patients in one by one.

Nita didn't know why they were there. Nobody had explained it to her. She just knew that a nurse came and got her from the workshop, told her to wash her hands and comb her hair, and took her to the conference room.

The young woman with the clipboard smiled when Nita came in. It was a real smile, not the tight professional smile the nurses wore. It made Nita nervous. In her experience, unexpected kindness usually meant something bad was about to happen.

"Hello, Nita," the woman said. "My name is Lois. These are my colleagues, Dr. Morrison and Mrs. Bowers. We're here to talk to you about your future."

Your future. What an odd phrase. Nita didn't have a future. She had a present that looked exactly like her past and would presumably continue until she died.

Lois pulled out a folder thick with papers. Nita's file. Seventy years of medical notes, incident reports, medication logs. A whole life reduced to paper and bureaucracy.

"We're from the Community Integration Program," Lois explained. "We're looking at patients who might benefit from living outside the hospital. In supervised residential settings. With support."

Nita didn't understand. Outside the hospital? She'd been here so long that the idea of anywhere else was almost incomprehensible and a bit fearful. How could she be somewhere where Nita didn't understand. Outside the hospital? She had been here so long that the idea of living anywhere else was hard to imagine and a little frightening. How could she manage in a place where no one told her what to do?

First Lois began to talk to her. "You work in the workshop. By all accounts, you're a model patient."

Mrs. Bowers, the older woman, spoke next. Her voice was gentle. "How would you feel about living in a house, Nita? With other people? With someone to help you, but more freedom than you have here?"

Freedom? Another strange word. Nita looked down at her hands, twisted and gnarled with arthritis. These hands that had carded thousands of sponges onto thousands of cards. These hands that had never held a phone, never turned a key in a lock, never done any of the ordinary things people did in the world outside.

"I don't know," she said quietly. It was the truth. She didn't know anything except this place.

They asked her questions. Simple ones. Could she dress herself? Yes. Could she shower without help? Yes. Could she follow simple instructions? Yes. Could she handle money? Nita hesitated. She had the forty dollars from the workshop, but she'd never actually spent money. Never been to a store. Never made a purchase.

"We can teach you," Lois said, seeing her hesitation. "That's what the program is for. To help people learn the skills they need to live in the community."

The interview lasted an hour. They were kind to her, these people from the outside. They treated her like she was a person who could make decisions, have opinions, want things. It was disorienting and wonderful and terrifying all at once.

After Nita left, the three of them sat in the conference room and went through her file more carefully. Admitted at age four for seizures. Parents never visited. No known living relatives. Seventy years in the same institution. Minimal life skills. Mind of a child in the body of an elderly woman.

"She's going to need a lot of support," Dr. Morrison said.

"She deserves a chance," Mrs. Bowers replied. "Seventy years. Can you imagine? Seventy years in this place when she was never dangerous, never violent, just a child with a medical condition that nobody understood."

Lois made a note in her folder. "I'll recommend her for placement. Let's see if we can find a host family who's up for the challenge."

Back on the ward, Nita sat on her bed and tried to imagine a house. A real house with rooms and windows that opened. She tried to imagine people who weren't nurses or patients. She tried to imagine a life that was different from this one.

The other patients noticed something had changed. Nita carried herself differently in the days after the evaluation. There was something in her eyes that hadn't been there before—not quite hope, but not complete resignation either. A possibility. A maybe.

Harold from the workshop asked her about it one day. "You seem different," he said in his precise, formal way. "Has something happened?"

Nita didn't know how to explain. How could she put into words this fragile, terrifying thing that was growing inside her? The possibility that she might leave this place. That she might have a different life. After seventy years of sameness, change felt both wonderful and impossible.

"Maybe," she said finally. "Maybe something good."

She started to notice things she'd stopped seeing long ago. The way the sunlight came through the high windows in the afternoon. The pattern of cracks in the ceiling above her bed. The sound of birds outside in the spring. These things had always been there, but Nita had taught herself not to notice them. Noticing meant caring, and caring about anything in here was dangerous.

But now she let herself notice. Let herself care. Because if she was leaving—and that was still a big if—she wanted to remember this place properly. Not just the bad parts, though those were many. But also the small kindnesses, the unexpected moments of beauty, the resilience of people who'd been broken but hadn't completely shattered.

But she couldn't. Decades of sameness had dulled her imagination. All she could picture was her bed, these walls, and the endless routine.

Still, something small and fragile had awakened inside her. Something that might have been hope, if she remembered what hope felt like.

Chapter 9: The Couple

Michael and Jenny Collins were thirty-two and thirty years old, respectively. They lived in a small house on Third Street with a fenced backyard and a garden that Jenny tended every evening after work. They had no children, but they'd fostered three dogs from the local rescue over the past five years.

When Lois from the Community Integration Program called them about Nita, Jenny had been hesitant. A person wasn't a dog. The commitment was bigger, the responsibility greater. But Michael, who worked as a teacher and believed deeply in giving people second chances, thought they should at least meet her.

They drove to the hospital on a Saturday morning. The buildings looked grim in the weak spring sunshine. The fence around the property made it look more like a prison than a place of healing. Jenny gripped Michael's hand as they walked to the main entrance.

Nita was waiting in the conference room, dressed in her best outfit—a simple dress that was too big for her small frame and shoes that had been polished by a helpful nurse. Her hair had been combed, her nails cleaned. She looked tiny sitting in the big chair, her feet barely touching the floor.

When Michael and Jenny came in, Nita looked up with eyes that were both hopeful and terrified. Lois made the introductions, explained the program, talked about expectations and support systems. But mostly, Jenny just looked at this small, elderly woman who'd spent seventy years in this place and felt her heart break a little.

"Hi, Nita," Michael said, sitting down across from her. "We heard you might be interested in coming to live with us for a while."

Nita nodded. She didn't know what else to do. These people seemed nice, but so had the visitors when she was four, and look how that had turned out.

"We have a spare bedroom," Jenny added. "It's small, but it has a big window that looks out on the garden. I grow tomatoes and beans and flowers. Do you like flowers?"

Nita had no idea if she liked flowers. She'd barely seen any in seventy years except through windows or on rare walks around the hospital grounds. "I... I don't know," she admitted.

Jenny smiled. "That's okay. We can find out together."

They talked for an hour. Michael and Jenny asked simple questions about what Nita liked to do, what she might want to learn. Nita answered as best she could, though most of her answers were "I don't know" or "I've never done that."

Before they left, Michael crouched down so he was at Nita's eye level. "If you decide you want to come stay with us, we'll do everything we can to help you. We know this is scary. We know you've been here a long time. But we think you deserve a chance to see what life is like outside these walls."

Nita felt tears prickling her eyes. Nobody had talked to her like this in... she couldn't remember how long. Like she mattered. Like her feelings mattered. Like she was a person, not just a patient.

"Yes," she whispered. "I want to come."

It took six weeks to process the paperwork. Six weeks of meetings and evaluations and training sessions. Lois met with Nita three times a week to teach her basic life skills. How to use a phone. How to lock and unlock a door. What to do in an emergency.

Nita was a good student, eager to learn. But some things were harder than others. The phone confused her. The sounds it made didn't seem connected to talking to people. The door locks required a kind of fine motor control her arthritic hands struggled with. And the whole concept of emergencies—that she could call someone for help—was so foreign to her experience that she couldn't quite grasp it.

But she tried. She tried so hard it made Lois want to cry sometimes. This woman who'd been given so little, who'd had seventy years stolen from her, was still willing to hope, still willing to try.

Finally, the day came. A sunny Tuesday in May. Michael and Jenny arrived with their car—Nita's first time seeing a car up close in seventy years. They loaded her few belongings into the trunk. A bag of clothes. Some toiletries. The forty dollars from the workshop. That was it. Seventy years reduced to one small bag.

Some other workshop patients lined up to say goodbye. Some of them had been there almost as long as Nita. They hugged her, wished her well. Harold from the workshop shook her hand formally, as if she were a colleague leaving a job. Mrs. Sauers, the head nurse, gave her a tight smile and told her to behave herself.

And then Nita walked out the front door of the hospital for the first time since she'd been four years old. The sunshine was so bright it hurt her eyes. The air smelled different—fresher, somehow. The sounds of birds and traffic and life were almost overwhelming after decades of institutional quiet.

Jenny took her hand. "Ready?" she asked.

Nita looked back at the stone building that had been her entire world. Then she looked at Jenny and Michael, these kind strangers who were willing to take a chance on her.

"Ready," she said.

The car ride was terrifying and wonderful all at once. Nita had forgotten what it felt like to move fast, to see the world rushing past the windows. Trees and houses and people living their ordinary lives. She pressed her face against the glass like a child, trying to take it all in.

Michael drove carefully, conscious of his precious cargo. Jenny sat in the back seat with Nita, pointing out things along the way. "That's the library," she said. "We can get you a library card if you'd like. Do you like to read?"

Nita had learned to read as a child in the hospital. The basics, anyway. But there weren't many books on the ward, and nobody had time to help her improve. "A little," she said quietly. "I'm not very good."

"We can work on that together," Michael said from the front seat. "I teach reading. It's what I do."

They pulled into the driveway of a small yellow house with white trim. It looked like the houses Nita had seen in picture books, the kind where families lived happy lives. She couldn't quite believe this was going to be her home now, even temporarily.

Michael came around and opened her door. This small gesture, opening the car door for her, made Nita's eyes fill with unexpected tears. In the hospital, doors were opened by whoever got there first. No one held them or waited. This simple kindness felt overwhelming.

Chapter 10: Learning to Live

The house on Third Street was small, but to Nita it seemed enormous. Rooms that led into other rooms. Stairs that went up to a second floor. Windows with curtains that you could open and close. A kitchen with appliances that hummed and beeped. It was all so much, so different from the ward.

Her room was upstairs, just like Jenny had said. A bed with a soft mattress and a quilt patterned with flowers. A dresser for her clothes. A window that looked out on the garden. Nita stood at that window for a long time, just watching the tomato plants sway in the breeze.

The first few days were the hardest. So many new things to learn. The bathroom had a shower, not a communal bath. The toilet flushed differently. There were light switches that controlled different lights. The front door had three different locks. Everything required explanation, demonstration, patience.

Michael and Jenny were endlessly patient. When Nita couldn't figure out how to work the toaster, Jenny showed her. When she didn't understand why the TV remote had so many buttons, Michael explained. When she asked the same questions over and over, they answered every time without frustration.

But there were challenges they hadn't anticipated.

The supermarket incident happened in the second week. Jenny took Nita shopping so she could learn where food comes from and be involved in the process. Lois, the social worker, had come along to help.

The supermarket was overwhelming. Bright lights. Hundreds of products. Music playing overhead. People rushing past with carts. Nita stayed close to Jenny, holding onto her arm like a child.

In the hospital, food had just appeared. Meals on trays, delivered at set times. Nita had never connected it with money, with choosing, with shopping. As far as she understood, things on shelves were just... there. Available. Free.

So, when she saw a package of cookies that looked good, she picked it up and put it in her pocket. Then a candy bar. Then a small bottle of juice. Jenny, busy reading a shopping list, didn't notice at first.

It was Lois who saw what was happening. Gently, she took Nita aside. "Nita, honey, we have to pay for these things. They're not free. We have to give the store money for them."

Nita didn't understand. Why did they have to pay? The things were just sitting there on the shelves. But Lois and Jenny were insistent. They had to put everything back. They had to pay for it first.

Frustrated and confused, Nita did what she'd learned to do in the hospital when things didn't make sense. She dropped to the floor and had a full-on tantrum. Lay there, kicking her feet. Refused to get up.

A seventy-four-year-old woman having a tantrum in the middle of the cereal aisle. People stared. Some whispered. A store manager came over, concerned. Jenny and Lois, mortified but understanding, tried to calm Nita down, tried to get her to stand.

It took twenty minutes before Nita was willing to get up, still not really understanding what she'd done wrong, but knowing from Jenny's face that she'd somehow messed up again.

They left the store without buying anything. Sat in the car for a long time while Lois explained again about money, about paying for things, about how stores worked. Nita tried to understand. She really did. But seventy years of institutionalization had left her without the basic framework that most people built in childhood.

That evening, sitting at the kitchen table, Jenny and Michael talked to Nita about other confusing things. The car door handle that Nita didn't know how to open from the inside. The concept of a gift—that you could give someone something they didn't have to pay you back for. The phone that she still couldn't quite understand.

Nita listened, tried to absorb it all. But it was so much. So overwhelming.

"I'm trying," she said, her voice small. "I'm trying so hard. But everything is different here. I don't know how to... how to be a person."

Jenny reached across the table and took Nita's gnarled hand. "You are a person," she said firmly. "You've always been a person. You just never got the chance to learn how to live in the world. But you're learning now. And we're going to help you."

The weeks passed. Slowly, things got a little easier. Nita learned to recognize which light switch controlled which light. She learned to ask before taking things. She learned that the car door handle pulled up, not pushed down.

Michael's birthday came in July. Jenny explained about gifts, about getting something special for someone you cared about.

They took Nita to the store—slowly, patiently—and told her she could choose something to give Michael.

Nita walked through the aisles, overwhelmed by choices. What did people want? What was special? In the hospital, nobody had wanted anything except to get out. She had no framework for this.

Then she saw it. In the refrigerated section. Bacon. Half a pound, wrapped in plastic. She remembered bacon from somewhere far back in her memory. Her mother cooking it on Sunday mornings. The smell filling their small kitchen. It was one of her few good memories from before.

She picked up the bacon and brought it to Jenny. "This," she said. "For Michael."

Jenny's first instinct was to redirect her. Raw bacon wasn't really a gift. But then she saw Nita's face, so earnest, so proud of having made a choice. She saw Lois watching from nearby, giving her a meaningful look that said: *Let her do this.*

"Okay," Jenny said. "Let's get it wrapped up nice."

They asked the butcher to wrap the bacon in brown paper and tie it with string, like a real present. Nita carried it carefully all the way home, protective of this thing she'd chosen, this gift she was giving.

At home, they kept it in the refrigerator. On Michael's birthday, when he opened the carefully wrapped package of raw bacon, he didn't laugh. He didn't look puzzled or patronizing. He just smiled and thanked Nita sincerely, telling her he'd cook it for breakfast the next morning.

And he did. He made bacon and eggs for all three of them, and they sat at the kitchen table together, and for the first time in seventy years, Nita felt like part of a family.

It wasn't perfect. She still had episodes where she didn't understand things. Still moments of confusion and frustration. She still sometimes dropped to the floor when overwhelmed. People in town whispered when they saw her, this strange old woman who didn't know how to work a doorknob, who acted like a child.

But she had her room with the window. She had Jenny teaching her about tomatoes and Michael reading to her in the evenings. She had Lois visiting twice a week and a new workshop in the community to attend. Everyone was patient and encouraging. She had people who saw her as a person, not a patient number. She even got to pick out the clothing she wore each day.

One evening, sitting in the garden as the sun set, Jenny asked her if she was happy.

Nita thought about it. Happy was such a big word. She didn't know if she understood it fully. But she knew that her feet hurt less here than in the hospital. She knew that nobody had put her in a quiet room. She knew that people talked to her, listened to her, treated her like she mattered.

"I think so," she said finally. "Yes. I think I might be happy."

It wasn't the ending she should have had. She should have had parents who understood seizures were medical, not demonic. She should have had a childhood, an education, a life. Seventy years shouldn't have been taken from her.

But this was the ending she had. A small room with a window. A garden with tomatoes. Two people who were patient with her confusion, kind about her limitations, determined to help her learn what it meant to live, really live, after so many years of just existing.

The learning continued every day. Small victories that most people took for granted. The day Nita successfully made toast all by herself. The day she answered the phone when it rang and managed to take a message for Michael. The day she remembered to turn off the bathroom light without being reminded.

Jenny started taking her to the garden. Showed her how to water the plants, how to pull weeds, how to tell when a tomato was ripe. Nita's arthritic hands made the work difficult, but she loved it anyway. Loved the smell of the earth, the warmth of the sun on her face, the simple satisfaction of helping something grow.

One day, after weeks of practice, Jenny let Nita pick a tomato herself. A perfect red one, warm from the sun. Nita held it in both hands like it was precious. In seventy years, she'd never grown anything, never been responsible for nurturing something from seed to fruit. This tomato felt like a miracle.

They cut it up for lunch, and Nita tasted fresh tomato for the first time she could remember. The sweetness exploded on her tongue, so different from the pale, tasteless slices served in the hospital cafeteria. She started to cry, overwhelmed by the simple goodness of it.

"It's okay," Jenny said, putting an arm around her shoulders. "Happy tears are allowed here."

The neighbors slowly got used to Nita. Mrs. Dowling next door started waving when she saw Nita in the garden. Mr. Mahew from across the street stopped looking confused when Nita didn't know how to respond to his "good morning" and started just smiling and going on his way. The mail carrier learned that Nita didn't understand about junk mail and started just handing Jenny the letters when she was home.

Not everyone was kind. Some people in town stared. Some whispered. Some said things Jenny and Michael would hear about later—that it was inappropriate, that woman living with them. That she should be in a home. That she was too damaged, too far gone, that trying to integrate her into normal life was cruel rather than kind.

But Jenny and Michael had learned to tune out the critics. They saw what others couldn't—the small daily triumphs, the gradual unfolding of a personality that had been locked away for seven decades. They saw Nita laugh for the first time at something funny on TV. They saw her choose her own clothes from the donations they'd gotten from the church. They saw her becoming, slowly but surely, a person who had choices and preferences and opinions.

Lois continued her visits, monitoring progress, offering guidance. One day, six months after Nita's arrival, she pulled Jenny and Michael aside.

"You know this is supposed to be temporary," Lois said gently. "The program is designed for placement, then transition to independence or other long-term care."

Jenny and Michael exchanged a look. They'd been thinking about this. Nita wasn't going to achieve independence—her cognitive limitations and age made that impossible. But the thought of moving her somewhere else, to another institution or group home, felt wrong.

"What if she just... stayed?" Michael asked. "What if this became permanent?"

Lois smiled. She'd been hoping they'd say that. "I'll start the paperwork," she said.

That evening, they told Nita. She'd been nervous all day, sensing that something important was being discussed. When they explained that she could stay, that this was her home for as long as she wanted it to be, she didn't quite understand at first.

"You mean... *forever*?" she asked, the word strange in her mouth. Forever was a concept that had meant something different in the hospital. Forever was punishment, endless days, time without meaning.

"Forever," Jenny confirmed. "Or for as long as you want. This is your home, Nita."

Nita looked up at the sky, darkening to purple as the stars began to appear. She was seventy-four years old, and she was just beginning to learn who she might have been, who she still might become.

It was a start. After seventy years, it was finally, impossibly, a start.

About the Author

P.A. Farrell writes accessible fiction that resonates with readers. Her work focuses on authentic human experiences and the quiet resilience of ordinary people facing extraordinary challenges. She is an accomplished flash fiction author whose compelling micro-narratives have captivated readers across the literary landscape. With over forty publications in prestigious online journals and literary magazines, Farrell has established herself as a master of the abbreviated form, crafting complete worlds and complex emotions within the constraints of brief word counts.

Her expertise in flash fiction extends beyond individual pieces to comprehensive collections, where she shows remarkable range and consistency in delivering powerful, bite-sized stories that linger long after the last sentence. Each collection showcases her ability to explore diverse themes, characters, and settings while maintaining the precision and impact that define exceptional flash fiction.

Farrell's work also resonates with readers who appreciate literature that delivers maximum emotional and intellectual impact in minimal space. Her stories often examine the pivotal moments that define the human experience, capturing the essence of larger truths through carefully chosen details and expertly crafted prose. The breadth of her publication history speaks both to her prolific output and the consistent quality that editors and readers expect from her work.

Through her continued contributions to the flash fiction genre, P.A. Farrell has become a trusted voice for readers seeking literature that respects their time while enriching their understanding of the human condition. Her collections offer the perfect opportunity to experience the full range of her storytelling abilities in a single, cohesive volume.

In her other life, P. A. Farrell is a clinical psychologist who has written several self-help books and continues to contribute to media outlets such as Medium.com and bluefly.com, where she posts articles on all aspects of healthcare, mental health, and a variety of other topics. Her Author's Page is here: https://tinyurl.com/4ewdunb8

Books by P. A. Farrell

Snowbound Hearts
The Secrets We Keep
The Secrets We Keep 2
Whispers Across the Sea
Love by the Latte
Echoes of Expectation—Waiting
Unexpected Short Tales of Surprise

A Special Request

If this book has touched your heart, sparked your curiosity, or simply entertained you along the way, I'd be incredibly grateful if you could take a moment to share your thoughts with a review on Amazon or wherever you discovered this book. Your words not only help other readers find books they'll love, but they also mean the world to authors like me who pour their hearts into every page. Thank you for being part of this journey, and for helping stories find their way to the readers who need them most. Her Author Page on Amazon: https://tinyurl.com/4ewdunb8

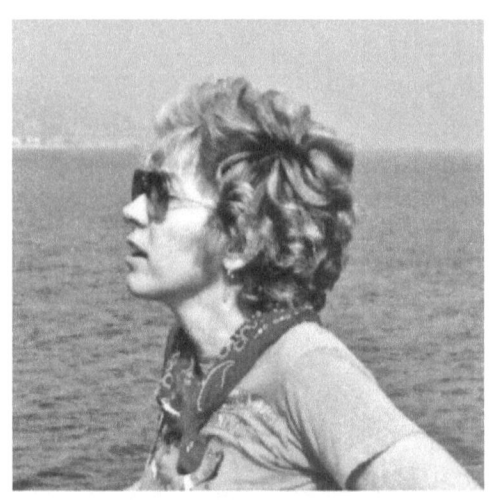

About the Author

P. A. Farrell is a psychologist and published author with McGraw-Hill, Springer Publishing, Cafe Lit, Ravens Perch, Humans of the World, Active Muse, Free Spirit Publishing, Scarlet Leaf Review, 100 Word Project, Woodcrest Magazine, Confetti, and LitBreak. She's a top health writer for Medium.com, has published self-help books, and is a board member of Clinics4Life. She lives on the East Coast of the US.

Read more at www.drfarrell.net.